TRUTH, LIES & ALZHEIMER'S ITS SECRET FACES

THE UNCONVENTIONAL PATH TO PEACE OF MIND FOR FAMILIES FACING ALZHEIMER'S AND DEMENTIA

LISA SKINNER

First Edition published under the title,

"Not All Who Wander Need Be Lost" - 2015

Printed in the United States of America

ISBN 978-1-0879-7596-2 (sc)

ISBN 978-1-0879-7600-6 (e)

Published by LISA SKINNER PRODUCTIONS

Contents

INTRODUCTION

A renowned entertainer once said that magic is "just spending more time on something than anyone else might reasonably expect." He was talking about creating magic in the entertainment industry. I work in a far less glitzy business - the eldercare industry. But I smile when I read the quote because a client of mine once remarked to me, marveling at how much better equipped he felt to manage his father's dementia symptoms, "What are you, some kind of Alzheimer's wizard?"

The truth is, I've just spent a lot of time working with families facing Alzheimer's and dementia related illnesses. I know what works and what doesn't. I've also lost family members to the disease. My years of experience are distilled into the chapters in this book. Each story contains a "further thoughts" section which explains how the symptoms, behaviors, and solutions from my experiences can apply to yours.

Learning to cope with brain disease is a lot like learning sign language if your loved one loses their hearing. At first you may feel overwhelmed and fearful that you'll never be able to communicate with them again. But with a little education, diligence, and practice you find a new way. The solution didn't involve your loved one getting their hearing back. Rather, it involved learning a new set of tools that allowed you to return to what mattered, enjoying your time spent with them.

My hope is that this book will vastly improve your ability to manage the challenging symptoms and behaviors associated with brain disease. Losing a loved one to Alzheimer's or dementia is one of the biggest challenges you'll ever face, but there is hope. The journey will be tough, and you'll have to learn some new skills. But by utilizing the tools in these chapters you can resume spending quality time with your loved one, and that's the real magic.

A Primer on Alzheimer's & Dementia-Related Illnesses

RT HERE

To understand dementia and its related behaviors, you have to understand what is happening to the brain of the person with dementia

Dementia is not a specific illness.

There are over 50 known causes of dementia, and most of them are irreversible.

Dementia is like a major organ failure.

Similar to heart or kidney failure - The affected organ with dementia is the brain.

imer's disease

umber one cause of dementia.

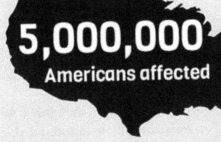

5,000,000

Americans affected

This number is expected to rise as the "Baby Boomer" generation begins to reach 65, according to the Alzheimer's Association.

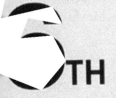

TH leading cause of death in the United States.

500,000 people a year die from **Alzheimer's disease.**

ementia is

rsistent loss of ectual functions ue to a brain disorder.

People typically lose their **recent memories** first.

It is a progressive disease.

Symptoms grow worse over time, progressing at different rates and stages.

Symptoms can be

d, moderate, or severe.

Not everyone displays every symptom

BIRDS IN THE MATTRESS

"Mrs. Walker is a nut. You need to do something with her," I over-heard the police officer say to my mother.

I was incensed. I wanted to scream at the officer: "My grandma's not crazy! She needs help." But I kept quiet. In those days you didn't talk back to adults, especially police officers.

I was a teenager, and it was just a few months after Nana told me about the birds in her mattress.

"What do you mean there are birds in your mattress?" I asked.

"They peck at my face at night," Nana responded.

What's wrong with my grandma, I thought. I wanted desperately to believe her. But what she was saying sounded impossible. Still, I checked the mattress on her bed, inside and out.

"I don't see anything, grandma. How are they getting in?"

"Oh, they're very clever," said Nana.

I went home and told my mom, who had already heard about the birds in the mattress. My mom revealed that Nana also thought people were stealing her jewelry, and that she refused to take showers because she was convinced "the men would come and kill her."

"Why didn't you say anything?" I asked my mother.

1

She looked down and took a drag from her cigarette, but remained silent. In those days you didn't talk about mental illness.

Over the next several months the behaviors worsened. Nana called the police several times a day to report the birds, the thieves, and the men who were going to kill her.

The trouble came to a head one day when Nana was driving to the store and became so disoriented that she stopped in the middle of a four-lane street, got out of her car and started wandering around.

A concerned citizen saw her and called the police, who called my mom and took Nana home. It was later that afternoon, back at Nana's house, where the officer scolded my mom, and called Nana a nut in front of us.

The incident prompted my mother to take Nana to a doctor, who diagnosed her with senile dementia, which is synonymous with today's Alzheimer's diagnosis. Nana was placed in a board and care facility where we visited her regularly until her death.

I still think about the officer who called my Nana crazy, and I can still recall the anger I felt toward him. But now that I have experience with the disease I see his comment through a different lens. After all, it's been 40 years. And dismissing her as a nut was his reaction to his unfamiliarity with brain disease.

As much as I would like to, I can't go back in time and change the police officer's mind about my grandmother being crazy. But moving forward, I can honor my grandmother's memory by educating people about the disease. She was my first experience with Alzheimer's, and the need I felt to help her still drives me today.

Further thoughts:

As was evident in this story, Mrs. Walker was experiencing delusions, hallucinations, and paranoia, which are not uncommon behaviors. You can see them displayed individually and separately, as you did in this story. Mrs. Walker's belief that there were birds living in her mattress and that they pecked her face at night is an example of a hallucination, which is a false sensory perception which usually manifests as hearing voices or seeing things which aren't there.

Believing that "the men were going to kill her in the shower" is an example of a delusion, which is a false belief. Mrs. Walker's belief would also qualify as a paranoid delusion because she believed someone was going to harm her. Unfortunately, no amount of reasoning can talk the person experiencing the delusion out of their belief. Often the most effective solution is to attempt to re-direct their attention to something else.

Finally, paranoia is often seen in those suffering from dementia. According to the Alzheimer's Association, approximately one out of three Alzheimer's disease sufferers will develop paranoia or suspiciousness. Many times a person with dementia will misplace a belonging and accuse someone else of taking it.

Because people with brain disease suffer from impaired reasoning, they may easily misinterpret others' intentions, and have difficulty understanding what is communicated to them. Their ability to separate fact from fiction may also be impaired.

Hallucinations, paranoia, and delusions can sometimes be mitigated with behavior management therapies. However, extreme psychotic symptoms may require medication. Establish a relationship with your loved one's doctor, and make sure the doctor is provided with consistent updates on your loved one's condition.

AULD LANG SYNE

When Julia found Sam, curled into a fetal position in his bed at the assisted living facility, he hadn't spoken in a year.

She had just opened a new memory care section at the facility where Sam was living. She was looking for residents who might do well in a more structured environment. She had read Sam's file, spoken to his caregivers, and had a hunch there was more life in him than they gave him credit for.

Sam had been at the assisted living facility for a few years. Without any family or friends to visit with, he had begun to withdraw, and spent most of his time in his room. Staff misinterpreted his decreased social engagement as a decline in health. They started bringing him all of his meals in bed and didn't encourage him to socialize. Shortly after that he stopped talking.

"I feel like Sam could vastly improve in a new environment. I think he's a good candidate for my program," Julia said.

Julia's strategically planned program kept residents engaged in activities based on their interests. Knowing that Sam, a WWII vet, had been a singer during the war, she encouraged him to go piano concerts held at the facility each week.

Just as Julia believed it would, Sam's condition vastly improved. Several months into his stay, Julia heard a story from a staff member that would melt her heart, and confirm her choice to bring him in.

The employee reported that Sam had been quietly sitting in the audience listening to the concert. On this day, during a particularly spirited singing of the classic "Auld Lang Syne," Sam stood up, leaned against his chair, and in sync with the other participants belted out the words to the chorus.

"Should old acquaintance be forgot, and never brought to mind. Should old acquaintance be forgot, and auld lang syne?"

A couple days later Sam walked in to Julia's office and sat down in front of her desk.

"Don't you look like the picture of perfect health," Julia said.

"I like it here," Sam responded.

Sam's health continued to get better, and he became more and more social with staff and the other residents.

Julia cried as she told me Sam's story, and I've re-told it countless times as an example of how all dementia care facilities are not created equal, and why environment matters.

Further thoughts:
In Sam's story, it is important to remember what caused the changes in his ability to communicate. I don't want to offer false hope to my readers that Alzheimer's and dementia related illnesses are reversible. On the contrary, they are progressive, degenerative disorders that worsen over time.

Sam's initial caregivers mistook his decreased social engagement for a decline in cognitive health. This caused him to spiral further into social isolation. The resurgence of his communication skills can be attributed to the new memory care program, which employed well-trained staff and utilized activities that tapped into Sam's basic need to feel like he belonged.

The right treatment environment can provide a sense of purpose and belonging. A big part of the solution is identifying activities that patients enjoyed during their primes. Helping them engage in those activities does wonders for their self-esteem, and provides much needed sensory stimulation. A well-coordinated program which incorporates these elements can decrease challenging behaviors, and most importantly, fulfills the patients' need to feel like they're living a meaningful life.

THE STRANGER
IN THE MIRROR

Nancy was sitting in the living room watching TV when she noticed Harold ambling down the hallway. He paused as he passed the hallway mirror, nodded at his reflection, and continued into the living room.

"Who's that guy?" he asked.

"What guy?" Nancy said.

"The older guy in the hallway."

Nancy looked down the hallway and saw the mirror.

"Oh, that's Harold," she said wryly.

"Oh," Harold said, shrugging, and then heading into the kitchen.

Over the next several months Nancy watched Harold's relationship with the new friend blossom. Nancy overheard Harold discussing a myriad of subjects with his friend including sports, aviation, and Harold's favorite kind of cookie – Lorna Doones.

"You've gotta try these," Nancy overheard Harold saying to the mirror one night. The next morning she found two smashed-up Lorna Doone cookies on the floor beneath the mirror.

One day Harold dashed into the living room and demanded to know where his reading glasses were.

"I didn't take your glasses," Nancy said without looking up from the TV.

Moments later she heard Harold's voice from the hallway. "You didn't take em, did ya buddy? Nah, you're not that kind of guy. I think you're my friend."

On another afternoon, Nancy caught her husband looking at his feet in the mirror. He turned to her and said, "Harold and I must be getting close. Apparently I gave him my shoes."

Nancy mentioned her husband's imaginary friend at an Alzheimer's support group she attended. She learned that Harold's behavior was a common phenomenon called "Stranger in the Mirror." She joked that Harold's new friend wasn't the stranger – it was her husband that she no longer recognized.

As Alzheimer's disease progresses, she learned, the short-term memory diminishes, and the person with dementia believes they are a younger version of themselves. When Harold looked in the mirror he saw an older man who couldn't possibly be him.

The group's recommendation was that she cover up the mirrors, or continue to "join his reality" by going along with his story.

Nancy went home that evening and covered up the mirror. "Mirror Harold" must have found a new place to hang out because Harold never mentioned him again.

Further thoughts:

The phenomenon of Stranger in the Mirror is an example of a hallucination, a common behavior seen with dementia. In Harold's story, the behavior ended up being relatively harmless. In fact, Nancy found the situation entertaining, and Harold had fun with his new imaginary friend.

However, in other cases, people can be frightened by the hallucination or even perceive it as a threat. For example, it is not uncommon for a person with dementia to walk into a bathroom, see themselves in the mirror, perceive their reflection as being a stranger, and refuse to take a shower.

As long as the individual suffering from the hallucination is not at risk of harming themselves or others, simply removing or covering up the mirror is an effective solution.

THE BEDROOM LITIGATOR

A thin layer of sweat shone from Tom's forehead as he made his way down the dementia unit hallway. He was desperately searching for something. He let out a muffled grunt as he lifted his walker, turned 90 degrees, and looked down a corridor adjacent to the hallway. A bead of sweat rose between his brow and temple.

"What's wrong Tom?" asked Sheila, calling to him from the nurses station.

"I can't find my God Damn office," Tom said, panicked.

"Oh, honey — you don't have an office no more. Go back to the dining room with your friends."

Tom, clearly agitated, snapped back, "Shut up, you don't know what you're talking about," and continued down the hallway.

Tom had been obsessed with getting to "work" every weekday morning for the past four months. Staff tried nearly everything to redirect him. But he was dogged and determined, just as he had been during his career as one of Washington D.C.'s top litigation attorneys. He was convinced he was needed at his office.

Louise, the facility's memory care director, had recently attended a conference on a new approach to treating the neurotic behaviors associated with brain disease called Reminiscence therapy. Reminiscence therapy is the re-creation a patient's personal environment as a scene they would recognize from their past.

With help from Tom's family, Louise re-created Tom's bedroom in the dementia unit to look like his office from when he practiced law.

The experiment worked. Every day after breakfast, Tom would say, "OK, I have to go to work now," and disappear into his "office" until evening. Staff members checked on him regularly and were pleased to see he was working diligently at his desk. Family members visited him and were relieved to see he was no longer agitated. The Reminiscence therapy had completely changed his behavior.

Treatments like Reminiscence therapy help patients cope with the loss of their core selves. For the young and resilient, it's often possible to recover from losing one's role in the world. Like a professional athlete whose career ends at age 30, we have the ability to face the reality of our situation and get to work redefining ourselves.

But that's not always possible for those afflicted with dementia. Brain disease robs them of the mental and physical resources required for that transition.

For Alzheimer's patients like Tom, the best we can do is keep them safe, engaged and comfortable in the last years of their lives. Treatments like Reminiscence therapy alleviate the uncertainty of shedding the skin of their former selves, and provide a smooth transition into the next, and often final stage of their lives.

Further thoughts:

This story is an example of common behaviors that can be triggered when a person's short-term memory is so diminished that they become disoriented to time and place, and believe they are living in a different period of their life. Tom's disease also led to personality changes such as irritability, anxiety, obsession with an idea that wasn't real, becoming easily angered, and aggression.

The caregivers' solution diffused Tom's behaviors and allowed him to re-engage with his surroundings in a calm and positive way. Because Tom's short-term memory was almost completely erased at this stage of the disease, there was nothing anyone could do to convince him that he lived in a dementia care facility, and no longer had a career and an office. Trying to change his reality would have been futile for his caregivers, and it would have only exacerbated the situation.

Success in Tom's story was about finding a creative way to "join his reality." Your loved one may have a different preoccupation. But the lesson is that with a little insight into what's driving that preoccupation, and a little creative troubleshooting, you can find a way to put your loved one at ease.

A DIVIDED FAMILY

It had been a long day at the office and I was finishing up some paperwork before heading home. From my desk, I could see our residents filing into the hallway and walking toward the auditorium where a concert was being held that night.

Two of the residents, both women, looked livelier than the rest. They stepped in tandem as they walked, snapping their fingers together to the same imaginary beat. One of the women stepped behind the other and placed her hands on her friend's hips, and they playfully rocked back and forth as they continued forward.

I did a double take when I realized who the woman in back was.

It was Anne.

I smiled as I recalled how much effort it had taken to get her here, and how worried two of her kids had been about whether this was the right environment.

Anne had four adult children. The two girls — Beth and Ellie — were adamantly opposed to putting their mother in the memory care section of the assisted living facility. Convincing them that mom needed to be in a professional environment felt like climbing Mount Everest with a 50 pound pack.

In most cases, if someone calls me it means they already have an open mind about getting help for their loved one. This case was unique in that Anne's two sons — Mark and Steve — had called to explore the options, but wouldn't commit without consensus from their sisters.

"I could never do that to my mother," Ellie insisted during our initial family meeting.

Anne had been living with her sister Kathy, and an incident that had occurred the week prior had convinced Beth and Ellie to at least attend the meeting.

Anne had taken Kathy's dog Kibbles for a walk — like she did every morning. Fifteen minutes later, Kathy was ironing her clothes when Kibbles came running into the house with her leash dragging behind her across the floor.

Kathy was heading out to look for her sister when her neighbor Bernadette called.

The neighbor had seen Anne trudging through her flower garden and went out to see if she could help.

"She didn't recognize me, and she didn't know where she was," Bernadette said.

This type of behavior was becoming more and more common with Anne. Less and less of what she said made sense. She was constantly saying she had to get somewhere, but could never articulate where she needed to go.

The Kibbles incident should have been the breaking point. But Beth and Ellie still wouldn't be convinced that a change was needed for their mother. Their stubbornness wasn't uncommon for Baby Boomers whose parents grew up fearing the institutionalization of the 1920s. For these adult children, there was often an unspoken understanding to avoid "putting their parents away."

In the end, it was Kathy who got Beth and Ellie to change their minds. During a family meeting, Kathy broke down and in a tear-filled admission said she could no longer meet the demands of being her sister's caregiver. Her heartfelt plea caused Beth and Ellie to rethink their insistence on keeping their mom out of a professional care environment.

I empathize with a family's desire to be loyal to their loved ones. In this case, Beth and Ellie didn't want to feel like their mom would be forgotten. They didn't want to feel like she would be "put out to pasture" — to live the rest of her life isolated and lonely. But their fears were steeped in a lack of education about the disease.

First, Alzheimer's and dementia patients thrive in environments where their minds are engaged. That is almost never the case when parents live at home —— or in Anne's case, with her sister. At Kathy's house, Anne spent most of her time on the couch watching TV. With little stimulation, it was no surprise that Anne's symptoms were progressing.

Second, many of today's eldercare facilities provide state-of-the-art care, utilizing evidence-based methods geared toward optimizing patient health. We've all heard stories about facilities that neglect or abuse residents. You can avoid those by knowing what to look for. For the most part, there's no better environment for a person suffering from brain disease — both in terms of treatment and safety — than an eldercare facility with a well-trained staff.

Beth and Ellie's resistance was ultimately a reflection of their own fear of deserting their mother. Unfortunately, their loyalty had created a potentially dangerous situation. It took a critical incident for them to realize their mother needed to be in the hands of professionals.

Further thoughts:

Anne getting lost while taking Kibbles for a walk is an example of wandering, one of the most common behaviors seen with Alzheimer's and related dementias. People with dementia wander for many reasons, including curiosity, because they are seeking companionship, or simply as a way of occupying their time. Wandering itself isn't a negative behavior if done in a safe environment. But as we saw in this story, wandering put Anne in danger because she was able to leave the security of her home, and then couldn't communicate who she was or where she was supposed to be.

In this story, we also witnessed some of the intense emotions family members feel while dealing with the behaviors and symptoms of the disease. Anger and frustration are very common. These emotions are usually an unconscious response to not knowing how to handle a situation, and/or fears associated with losing the loved one. Family members may also deny the existence of the disease and its symptoms; again, a coping mechanism for dealing with the uncertainty of the situation.

Family members may also feel guilty about surrendering control of their loved one's care to professionals. Even though they may know it logically, it may be hard for them to accept emotionally that trained caregivers can provide the safety and stimulation that will allow their loved one to thrive.

SUNDOWNING

"You have to take me to find the house," Steve heard over the phone.

It was Jack, his dad, who called every night at 5:00 p.m. He sounded panicky. Steve didn't know which house his dad was referring to, and he never did ask.

Dad got a little confused from time to time, but he was fine, thought Steve.

The rest of the family begged to differ. Especially Steve's younger sister, Alice, who insisted that Jack should no longer live alone.

Alice had been researching Alzheimer's symptoms, and explained that the agitation and confusion their dad was experiencing every night was called sundowning. She had researched local eldercare facilities and told Steve that living in one could improve their father's quality of life.

Steve wouldn't listen. His dad, born during the depression, had been placed in an orphanage at eight years old. For men of Jack's era, institutionalization was synonymous with abandonment. In fact, Jack had once told his son, "I'd rather have you put a gun to my head and pull the trigger than put me in one of those homes."

Steve remained adamant. "I know how to take care of my own father," he said.

But the sundowning behaviors only got worse. Steve started receiving calls from a manager at the local Hooters restaurant, who complained that Jack was asking out the young servers.

17

"How old is your dad?" the manager asked.

"He's 84."

"Well, when he's in our restaurant he acts like he's 24. Can't you keep him at home?"

After the fourth call from the Hooters manager, Steve's sister Alice brought up the subject again.

Steve remained stubbornly opposed. "Dad doesn't need to go into a nursing home. I'll just keep setting him straight," he said.

It wasn't until Jack went missing for two days — and police officers found him sleeping in his car in the Hooters parking lot — that Jack conceded to getting help.

Alice found an opening at a local memory care facility. However, Steve believed his dad belonged in a less restrictive assisted living facility — and saw him as much higher functioning than the residents in the memory care unit.

"I can't put my dad in there with those crazies. He'll die," said Steve.

Fortunately, the eldercare facility's administrator was vocal in his belief that Jack needed to be in memory care. The administrator asked Steve to go on a tour of the facility. Steve was surprised to see that the residents looked happy; the facility even felt home-like.

Steve finally conceded to placing his dad in memory care.

When he visited his dad two weeks later, Steve was surprised to hear how well his dad was adjusting (aside from two incidents where he was given a time out for asking out the female wait staff).

In fact, during Steve's visit, Jack was so engaged in the facility's arts and crafts activity that he barely acknowledged his son.

Through talks with staff, Steve learned that "the house" his dad had been trying to find was the home he lived in before being placed in the orphanage. Jack no longer talked about trying to find "the house." He now bragged about his new chore at the facility — sweeping the back patio — which he did promptly every night at 5:00 p.m.

Further thoughts:

Sundowning refers to a set of behaviors, in which the person with dementia is disoriented and confused, typically occurring at the end of the day (although the behaviors can actually occur at any time). The person suffering from sundowning can experience dramatic changes in personality and behaviors including pacing, wandering, suspiciousness, disorientation, confusion, and agitation. The person may be demanding and combative, or yell out and scream for no apparent reason. The causes and triggers of sundowning are not clearly understood.

Another common behavior illustrated in our sundowning story is elopement. Elopement is different from wandering (which we saw in a previous chapter) in that the person has a specific destination in mind and is determined to find it. They typically seek to exit their current environment, and have a purpose or agenda to get somewhere. It is very common for a person with dementia to want to find a deceased spouse who they believe is worried about them. A person exhibiting sundowning behaviors can be relentless in their pursuit of what they are looking for. They may even believe they are being kept against their will and may become angry, anxious, and/or aggressive.

The most important thing to recognize about sundowning is that the behaviors and symptoms are part of the disease and not the intentional behavior of the person. The behaviors displayed when a person is sundowning can usually be effectively managed with assistance from a trained professional.

THE PILL BOX

I parked in front of Harvey and Darlene's house in the older part of Red Bluff, pausing for a moment to collect myself. I had to put my game face on.

This wasn't an ordinary assessment. I wasn't going in as Lisa Skinner, the eldercare advisor. I'd be posing as a friend of Darlene's daughter, Carly, who had called me to help with her dad. In our phone conversation Carly said her dad was, "totally out to lunch," and "couldn't do anything for himself."

I didn't want Harvey to know he was being assessed by a professional, so I asked Carly to introduce me as a friend. My plan was to have a casual conversation with him, even though I'd prepared questions to assess his cognitive ability.

Carly answered the door and walked me to the kitchen where Darlene was standing at the counter with a glass of wine, and Harvey was seated at the kitchen table.

"Mom, Dad — this is Lisa…," she said.

Harvey interjected, "Oh, you must be Carly's friend who's going … somewhere…"

This was clue number one. Carly had told her father I was stopping by on my way to the Shakespeare Festival in Ashland, Oregon, which my husband and I attended every year.

Harvey didn't remember where I was going, but he remembered that Carly's friend would be stopping by. Someone as far gone as Carly had described would not have retained that much information.

I sat down at the table and smiled at Harvey. I noticed a blue pill organizer on the windowsill marked "M T W TH F." I pointed and asked, "What's that?"

"That's my thing," he said.

"What does it do?"

"The things I put in there are the things that keep me alive."

Darlene snickered. I looked up to see her toss a sip of wine into her mouth.

Pretty early in the day for a glass of wine, I thought.

I remembered what Carly had told me about her mom and dad during our first conversation. Their marriage had been on the rocks before Harvey started showing signs of Alzheimer's. Now that his health was in decline she felt trapped.

I continued with Harvey, "Well how do you know where to put the things?"

He couldn't recall the word for medication, or what the letters on the organizer stood for. But he showed me how he took a pill from the prescription bottle and put it in the leftmost compartment, and then the next one to the right, and so on until he reached the end.

"The old codger gets em' right every time — I check," Darlene chimed in.

I paused for a moment to reflect. Suddenly the picture became clearer. Darlene resented Harvey because his disease was keeping her in an unhappy marriage — now a marriage where her role was changing to being his full-time caregiver. Darlene wanted to remain loyal, but the idea of having to do everything for her husband was daunting.

Carly, on the other hand, was mistaking her father's decline in verbal skills for a decline in cognitive skills.

This made sense based on what she had told me about their relationship. She used to call him to ask for advice on relationships, finances, etc. But she couldn't do that anymore because of his verbal decline. She missed being able to talk to him; she was mourning the loss of the man she grew up depending on. Perhaps in her mind it was easier to think of him as already gone, which would further explain why she described him as so incapable.

I continued my conversation with Harvey and his family, but in a way I had already completed my assessment.

I recommended that Harvey stay at home with Darlene, and gave her a list of activities to keep him engaged. I supplied a list of behaviors to look out for so they'd know when he started declining.

The experience was a reminder of the importance of having an objective assessment done by a professional. Carly and Darlene weren't intentionally misreading the signs —they were just viewing them through the lens of their own needs, fears and desires.

The changes I recommended were geared toward keeping Harvey as independent as possible, which of course Darlene was relieved to hear.

Further thoughts:

Harvey suffered from Aphasia, the loss of ability to communicate. There are many types of Aphasia, and it can present itself in several ways (Refer to the glossary for a list of types). The condition results from damage to the communication centers of the brain. The location and extent of the damage determines the type of Aphasia that is present.

During my assessment, it was evident that Harvey was very high functioning cognitively. He understood everything that was being said to him. However, he had difficulty finding the correct word to use, and articulating his thoughts. For example, when I asked him what the pill box was, he could not remember the correct name for it, even though he obviously knew its function. A more cognitively impaired person would not be able to recognize what a pill box was, and what it was used for, as Harvey did.

There were a lot of misperceptions from family members in this story. That's natural, and is no negative reflection on the family members. We all have blind spots, myself included. It's nothing to be ashamed of. I find my blind spots are worked out when I seek the opinion of people I trust, which often means consulting professionals.

FACE VALUE

"I don't take those behaviors at face value. Something else could be contributing to them," said Donna.

I felt relieved. "Whew, that's what I was hoping you'd say," I replied.

I was trying to place Esther, a difficult resident to say the least, into a new residential care home. She had already been turned down by two board and cares.

Esther was a night wanderer. In the current facility where she lived, she had walked into several residents' rooms in the middle of the night, scaring them half-to-death. She continually collected their belongings and hid them in different places in her room.

She was also what's known as a painter, and not because she requested a canvas and acrylics from staff. Several times in the last couple months she had taken off her diaper and smeared feces on the wall.

Her caregivers also reported that she was verbally combative, and would lash out when staff tried to redirect her.

The facility where she lived said it wasn't equipped to handle her behaviors, so Esther's son had called me to find her a new home.

Donna, an expert in dementia care who owned six facilities, saw the same thing I did when reading Esther's file: several issues that could be influencing her behaviors other than brain disease.

First, Esther had been prescribed an antipsychotic medication. While the medication itself wouldn't necessarily have caused the behaviors, it was possible that she was experiencing unpleasant side-effects, and was acting out in an effort to communicate her discomfort.

Second, Esther had a history of urinary tract infections, and she hadn't seen her doctor in several weeks. It was possible that she was experiencing pain from an infection, and her behavior was an attempt to communicate that.

Third, Donna and I both knew that the staff at Esther's current facility had very little dementia training. Also, for most of the care staff at this particular facility, English was not their first language. So it was possible that a gap in communication and training was increasing Ester's confusion and frustration.

"I'm going to accept Esther," said Donna. "I honestly believe we can turn some of these behaviors around once she sees her physician again and she's in the right environment."

And that's exactly what Donna did. Before admitting Esther to her facility, she scheduled an appointment with Esther's psychiatrist and primary care physician. The psychiatrist adjusted Esther's meds, and it turned out she did have a urinary tract infection.

Two weeks later I went to check on Esther in her new home. I walked into the facility and started to ask for Esther – but then I saw her. She was sitting on the couch in the living room with another female resident; both had their hands folded gently across their laps, and were calmly observing some of the other residents play a game.

"She's actually doing very well," said one of the caregivers. "She still has some incontinence problems, but there hasn't been any night wandering, or any of the other behaviors she came in with.

"On the contrary," she continued, "Esther now has a problem of her own." The caregiver described how Esther's new friend, seated next to her living room, had taken quite a liking to Esther, and followed her everywhere she went. Esther's son was also visiting often, and it seemed like they had a nice time when they were together, the caregiver said.

This story was told from my perspective as a professional eldercare advisor. But we all eventually find ourselves in a place where a loved one's behavior just seems "difficult," or even "crazy." Esther's story is an example of how we must, with the help of professionals, look for extenuating circumstances before drawing conclusions about how to manage symptoms.

Further thoughts:

This story exemplifies several behaviors that are common with dementia, including agitation and combativeness, wandering/nighttime walking, trailing, hoarding/collecting, and "painting."

It is important to understand that as Alzheimer's disease continues to destroy memory and mental skills, it also begins to alter emotions and behaviors. Approximately 70 to 90 percent of Alzheimer's patients eventually develop behavioral symptoms. Agitation is one of the most common behaviors seen with dementia, and can be displayed in a variety of ways, including restlessness, pacing, fear, and/or in changes in body language or facial expressions. Agitation can also easily escalate to aggression if not responded to appropriately. Individuals suffering from dementia will exhibit behaviors within a range of extremes. This is because the brain is attacked in different places and at different rates of speed, so each person's behaviors will be different (although a variety of identifiable behaviors are commonly seen).

A behavior should be considered a problem if it has a negative impact on the person afflicted or on others around him/her. The behaviors can be triggered by one or more of several contributing factors such as environmental issues like sensory overload, too much noise, or even the temperature of a room. It could also occur if a task is too overwhelming or complicated. It could also be a physical or emotional reason, as well as communication disconnect between the person and a caregiver. There are so many underlying reasons why a person might be reacting. The important thing is to keep in mind that the reactions, or behaviors, are the only way a person with dementia may be able to communicate that there is a problem that needs to be addressed.

That said, one of the most important principles of this chapter, Face Value, is just that: You have to be careful not to take the behaviors at face value or rush to judgment about what's causing them. Through process of elimination the underlying reason can be uncovered.

DOGGIE DEMENTIA

"Oliver!" …. "Oliver!!" my husband yelled from the front doorway of our home.

He was trying to get our 16-year-old Cockapoo to go outside to go to the bathroom.

But Oliver just stood there, with a deer-in-the-headlights look. He didn't know what he was supposed to do. It hadn't always been that way, of course. Oliver had been a smart, funny, energetic dog for most of his life.

I remember the first time I noticed a change in his behavior. We were at our house in the Sierra Nevada, which is one of his favorite places to go because he grew up there. But this time he didn't seem happy. He seemed anxious. And every few minutes he would get up from his dog bed and pace around the house.

Over the next year, his confusion and anxiety worsened. I took him to the vet and half-jokingly asked if dogs got dementia.

"As a matter of fact they do, but we don't call it that. We call it Canine Cognitive Dysfunction," said the veterinarian.

The vet said there wasn't much we could do to treat Oliver's symptoms. Since then, we've been doing our best to manage his behavior. A few times he's gone potty on the carpet. I initially think to myself, "He should know better," but then I remember it's the disease causing the behaviors and tell myself, "He's not trying to be a bad boy; he's trying to be a good boy. He's trying to please us."

We're all familiar with the saying "Don't kick the dog" — or, in other words, don't take your anger out on someone who's helpless and didn't intentionally hurt you. But I see a lot of "dog kicking" in families dealing with Alzheimer's and other dementia related illnesses. I see spouses acting resentful toward their partners, as if they blame their partners for getting brain disease.

These spouses find themselves in a difficult position: caregiver to a partner who can no longer fulfill his or her role. The very person they trusted to provide security and safety is now childlike and helpless. The important thing is to remind ourselves, as often as we need to, that the behaviors are not coming from the person we knew. It's a result of the disease, and what is happening to the brain.

If our goal is to appreciate the remaining time we have left with our loved ones, patience and understanding is required. It's not all that different from having an old dog who piddles on the carpet. Sometimes all you can do is laugh, forgive, and tell him he's a good boy.

Further thoughts:

Yes, dogs do get dementia! I wasn't trying to be funny or flippant by including a story about K-9 Cognitive Disorder in this book. I wouldn't want to diminish the experience of our friends and loved ones who suffer from brain disease. But I do want to raise awareness of some of the symptoms associated with dementia, regardless of whether they're exhibited by people or our pets. Many of us consider our pets family, so it can be painful to see them decline mentally as well.

Cognitive decline in dogs is similar to what we see in people. Canine Cognitive Dysfunction primarily affects memory, learning and comprehension. Brain function is affected by the physical and chemical changes that happen with the aging process. In dogs, there is no breed disposition. The dog's age is the biggest predictor.

Dogs affected by Canine Cognitive Dysfunction can exhibit the following symptoms/behaviors: Wandering and pacing, acting "dazed" or staring off into space, getting lost in familiar places, general confusion and disorientation, being restless for no apparent reason, not responding to commands they once knew, and becoming withdrawn or disinterested in daily activities.

Don't hesitate to take your pet to a doctor if they are experiencing similar symptoms. I'm grateful that my experience helping families facing brain disease allowed me to recognize similar symptoms in Oliver. I'm equally grateful that Oliver's veterinarian was educated in how to handle the disorder.

THE CHANGING
STATION

For about a month-long period while working at a memory care facility in Washington D.C., I dreaded giving family tours.

I was afraid of Martha's screams. Not that they signified an emergency; Martha was safe and in good hands.

I was afraid of what the families would think when they heard her screams.

I would be in the middle of giving a tour to a family who was considering trusting our staff to care for their loved one. And then from behind some closed door Martha would shriek like she was being eaten alive by zombies. I would try to reassure the families that her screaming was a behavior associated with the disease, but I was never sure if they believed me.

And the truth was, we didn't know what was wrong with Martha. She was physically healthy aside from her Alzheimer's diagnosis. She was just trying to communicate something, but we didn't know what it was.

During that time, I had been attending trainings on new evidence-based behavior modification strategies. An emerging approach was the placement of life-stations in memory care units. Life-stations are work-stations adorned with props for residents to play with. The props keep their brains engaged, and trigger positive memories from their past.

Many of our residents in the memory care unit had been stay at home moms, so I set up a life-station with a crib, bassinet, diaper changing table, a baby girl doll, and several changes of clothes.

About a week after setting up the station I noticed that I hadn't heard Martha scream in a while. I asked one of the caregivers about Martha.

"She's a completely different person, and you can take credit for that," the caregiver said. "She adopted the baby doll as her own, and never lets it out of her sight. And she hasn't screamed since."

So often when we talk about Alzheimer's disease, we focus on the effect it has on the family. Slowly losing our loved one to brain disease is one of the hardest things we'll ever face. But we speak as if our loved one is already gone — as if there's no longer a person in that body who's aware of his or her surroundings. And that's not always true.

Alzheimer's disease is often a double whammy for the afflicted. Not only do they lose their ability to make sense of their world, but also the ability to articulate their needs. Combine that with a changing — and confusing — environment, it makes sense that a person with Alzheimer's Disease would act out, which in Martha's case manifested as these horrible screams.

Martha was reacting to a new and uncertain environment in which she no longer knew her role. She had identified as a caregiver — a mother — for so long that the prospect of losing that role was overwhelming. Further, she didn't know how to articulate her need to have a purpose. Like a child who doesn't have the words to express concern, the best she could do was scream for help.

The life-station not only satiated Martha's need to nurture her maternal instincts, but it helped her transition to her new station in life — that of an Alzheimer's resident who could let herself be cared for by the caregiving staff.

Further thoughts

Martha's story is a prime example of someone whose challenging behaviors were an attempt to communicate a need. Your loved one may exhibit a different challenging behavior. For example, some people who suffer from Alzheimer's or dementia become combative during showers. This comes from a lack of ability to task sequence. The person suffering from brain disease believes the shower is finished, and attempts to communicate their belief by trying to stop you from finishing the shower.

Martha was trying to communicate a deep-seated need to be maternal. This is very different than someone whose brain disease prevents them from recognizing correct task sequence. But the similarity is that the individual suffering from the disease perceives a need. The need doesn't have to make sense or be rooted in reality.

The lesson we can learn from Martha is that sometimes it takes creative troubleshooting to identify an activity that fulfills a need, and thus allows the challenging behavior to subside. Try getting your loved one involved in different types of activities. Make sure they're safe. Your loved one's speaking ability may be impaired, so they won't be able to tell you if the activity is working. But you can read their non-verbal cues and identify activities that visibly put them at ease. By experimenting with activities that they naturally enjoy you can often put your loved one's challenging behaviors to rest.

MARYANNE

My mother-in-law, Maryanne, 83, was fidgeting with a tissue. As she often did, she folded it into a neat little square, and put it in her purse. Moments later she took it out, folded it again, and tucked it back into her purse.

Fold. Tuck. Repeat.

She was staying with us for the day while we gave her usual caregiver, my sister-in-law, a break.

Maryanne was sitting on the couch in the living room watching The Andy Griffith Show.

She looked peaceful. But it didn't last long.

She sat up suddenly; visibly anxious.

"Does Marty know where I am? You better take me home. He's going to want his dinner," she said.

Did she really just ask where Marty was, I thought. He'd been dead for four years.

It was hard for me to hear, even as a specialist in the field. I'd been helping families understand brain disease for years. But just like everyone else, I tended to react emotionally when it came to my own family.

My first instinct was to correct Maryanne. I saw how much her decline hurt my husband, and I wanted to pull her back into reality.

But I knew better. Joining her reality was the only way to diffuse the behavior.

"Yes, he knows you're here. I just called him. He knows I'll be bringing you home soon."

"Are you sure?" Maryanne said.

"Yes, I'm sure."

"Well, OK," said Maryanne. "I just don't want Marty to be worried."

She went back to watching The Andy Griffith Show. A couple minutes later she pulled out the tissue.

Fold. Tuck. Repeat.

She looked peaceful.

It hurt to fib to Maryanne. It still hurts when I think about it today.

But correcting her might have caused her to panic. In her mind, her husband was waiting at home. There's nothing anyone could have done to convince her otherwise. It would have been like she was hearing the news for the first time.

When a person's defenses are up, as Maryanne's would have been if we told her the truth, she wouldn't have been able to connect with us on an interpersonal level. Telling Maryanne the truth wouldn't have caused her to "snap out" of her belief. Believing that Marty was alive was her reality for the moment. By joining her reality, I relieved her concern, and ensured that we would continue to have an enjoyable visit.

The conflict I felt over stretching the truth was a fair trade for her peace, even if it was only temporarily. She would never be "normal" again. But there would be times where she would be OK; where we could still connect. Those were the moments I worked for.

Further thoughts:

As we saw in this story, people with dementia can seem perfectly fine one moment, and in the next they can be anxious and detached from reality. This can be one of the most troubling behaviors for families to deal with. The difficulty stems from not wanting to see our loved one uncomfortable, and from not knowing how to handle a problem that only exists in their mind.

Losing touch with reality is a normal progression of the disease. This is due to the short term memory diminishing throughout the course of the illness. You can think of the short term memory as if it were hooked up to a light fixture which can be switched on and off. In the earlier stages of the disease the switch stays on most of the time, but as the disease progresses the switch is sometimes on and sometimes off. In the end, the switch goes off permanently and the person's perception may be completely detached from reality.

Maryanne believed that her husband was still alive; your loved one will likely have a different false belief. Remember that no matter what you do you cannot dissuade the person of their belief. This is why "joining their reality" is the most effective approach. The essence of the approach is to acknowledge their reality, and then divert their concern. In Maryanne's case, this meant acknowledging that her husband was at home, but explaining why there was no reason to be worried. The situation with your loved one may be different, but you can use the "acknowledge and divert" approach to diffuse the situation.

Lastly, Maryanne also exhibited repetitive behaviors. Fold, tuck, repeat! Your loved one may repeat words, activities, questions, or stories. They may also pace around a room. These types of behaviors are often a coping mechanism for dealing with stress or fear. Admittedly they can be annoying for family members and caregivers. Do what you can to redirect them. But as long as the behaviors are safe, eliminating them isn't mission critical.

CONCLUSION

Thanks for taking the time to read about some of my experiences with Alzheimer's and dementia related illnesses. There's no getting around the difficulty of losing a loved one to brain disease. You may feel like you're losing your loved one twice: Once during their cognitive decline, and again with their physical death. You may feel like you're losing someone who you used to count on. You might not know what you're going to do when they're gone.

Knowing others have been there too won't make things normal again, but it may make your journey less daunting. Most people who lose someone they love want things to go back to the way they were; when things were simple, and when spending time with family was everything.

The families I described in this book found small ways to get back to that special place, and so can you. It may not be the "normal" you remember, but it can be a new normal. You can still enjoy the company of the one you love.

I hope the lessons contained in these stories can help get you back to that place. Don't hesitate to contact me if I can help along the way.

Sincerely,

Lisa Skinner

WHAT DOES DEMENTIA LOOK LIKE ON A DAY-TO-DAY BASIS?

The following is a list of signs and symptoms associated with common dementia behaviors. Alzheimer's disease and other dementias affect people in different ways. Each person will experience symptoms differently.

Aggression – Signs may include a hostile or destructive mental attitude or behavior, such as a harmful action towards another. Aggressive behaviors can be physical, such as hitting or pushing, or verbal, such as shouting, screaming, or name calling.

Agitation – Signs may include restlessness, fear, pacing, and different than normal body language and facial expressions.

Anger – Signs may include displeasure, resentment, indignation, and/or rage.

Anxiety – Signs may include irritability, depression, pacing, constant movement, restlessness and general emotional distress.

Apathy- Signs may include an absence of emotion or an absence of interest or enthusiasm for things generally considered interesting.

Aphasia –Signs may include the loss of ability to communicate, such as difficulty understanding and/or expressing spoken or written language. Aphasia may be mild or severe. With mild aphasia, a person may be able to converse, yet have trouble finding the right word or understanding complex conversations. Severe aphasia limits a person's ability to communicate. A person may say little and may not participate in or understand any conversation. There are many different types of aphasia including:

- **Anomic Aphasia** – A person may speak normally but has difficulty in articulating the name of an object or place;
- **Conduction Aphasia** – A person has trouble repeating words spoken by someone else; otherwise, speech is fairly normal;
- **Expressive Aphasia (Broca's aphasia)** – A person can hear and understand, but cannot express his/her own thoughts;
- **Fluent Aphasia** – A person speaks normally or rapidly, but may unconsciously substitute words or sounds with incorrect choices. They don't realize that they are making these errors, so they will not correct themselves. For example, they may say cat when they mean dog;
- **Global Aphasia** – A person has difficulty speaking, repeating, or comprehending language altogether;
- **Non-fluent Aphasia** – A person speaks slowly and with difficulty. He/she may grimace and use hand gestures in attempting to communicate. He/she may leave out words and endings of words when speaking;
- **Receptive Aphasia (Wernicke's aphasia)** – A person can hear what is said but cannot understand; they can speak, but cannot understand or monitor their own speech.

Catastrophic reaction – Signs may include hitting, yelling, running, or combativeness. It is an extreme emotional reaction that is out of proportion to the actual event. A catastrophic reaction occurs when a person is unable to communicate or articulate a need such as having to go to the bathroom, experiencing pain, or is the result of a frustrating situation that escalates. This behavior may occur suddenly without an apparent reason.

Communication difficulties – Signs may include the inability to properly communicate one's needs due to the effect dementia has on the brain resulting in problem behaviors. They may also include problems with word finding, putting one's thoughts smoothly into words, and the ability to understand written or verbal language. Most often the behaviors are triggered by frustration, anger, or agitation because a person doesn't understand what he/she is being asked to do and is unable to make themself understood.

Confusion – Signs may include losing track of dates, seasons and the passage of time. May include forgetting where they are or how they got there, or having trouble understanding something if it is not happening immediately.

Delusions – Signs may include believing in a false idea that is contrary to fact, and remaining persistent in that belief (ex: insisting that "you are not my son.")

Depressive behaviors – Signs may include impaired concentration, memory loss, apathy, lack of interest in formerly enjoyed activities, overwhelming sadness, crying more than usual, significant weight loss or gain, sleep disturbances or sleeping more or less than usual, restlessness, feelings of guilt or worthlessness, and/or talking less than usual.

Disorientation – Signs may include the inability to know one's place or time, such as not knowing the day of the week, the time of day, or getting lost in familiar places, and/or not recognizing familiar places or things.

Disorganized behavior – Signs may include bizarre or socially inappropriate behaviors such as undressing in public, screaming in public, or collecting unusual things, such as napkins.

Disrobing – Signs may include taking their clothes off at inappropriate times or places. May be a sign of discomfort or even boredom.

Eloping - Signs may include watching the exit doors, elevators, etc., in hopes of finding an opportunity to "escape" from their current surroundings.

Hallucinations – Signs may include false perceptions of objects or events that a person with dementia may see, hear, smell, taste, or feel something that isn't actually there, such as hearing someone talking who isn't there, or seeing insects crawling on walls that are not there.

Hoarding – Signs may include stockpiling, storing, or collecting items and placing them in a hidden or carefully guarded place for preservation, future use, etc.

Impaired concentration – Signs may include difficulty in paying attention and in staying on task.

Impaired judgment – Signs may include the inability to use reasoning skills in using judgment or decision making such as when it is safe to cross a street, or when dealing with money.

Impaired Visual Images and Spatial Relationships – Signs may include the inability to interpret what one sees, and to properly recognize objects, sounds, shapes, or people, even when eyesight is not impaired. A person may have difficulty reading, judging distance and determining color or contrast.

Inability to sequence tasks – Signs may include the inability to perform a skilled or learned task that requires putting together steps of a process, such as getting dressed or even taking a shower.

Inappropriate sexual behavior – Signs may be masturbating in public, disrobing, or attempting to have sex with an inappropriate person or thing. A person may mistake another person for their spouse.

Incontinence – Signs may include lack of control or involuntary urination or defecation.

Memory loss – Signs may include difficulty recalling recent events.

Misplacing things – Signs may include putting things in unusual places, misplacing objects and not being able to retrace their steps. Many times this results in accusing others of stealing.

Mood changes – Signs may include becoming confused, suspicious, depressed, fearful, anxious, and/or easily upset for no apparent reason.

Multiple layers of clothing – Signs include putting on multiple layers of clothing, such as three different sweaters, or several different pairs of pants, etc., at the same time.

Pacing – Signs may include excessive walking up and down a hallway, or in and out of a building, or around and around a building with no specific purpose.

Paranoia – Signs may include an unrealistic, blaming belief, such as unreasonable suspiciousness that someone has stolen something, or that someone is doing something that they are not.

Personality changes – Signs may be noticeable differences in personality, or exaggerated changes in normal personality characteristics.

Pocketing – Signs may include holding small bits of food between a person's cheek and gums.

Poor table manners – Signs may include mixing, stirring, pouring, not using utensils, using inappropriate condiments, etc., due to not recognizing or remembering the proper ones.

Psychosis – Signs may include hallucinations, delusions, and/or paranoia.

Repetitive Behaviors – Signs may include saying or doing something over and over again, such as repeating words, questions, or activities.

Rummaging – Signs may include searching through something in order to find an object of interest, often causing disorder and/or confusion.

Sleep disturbances – Signs may include sleeping more or less than usual, interrupted sleep patterns, and/or unusual sleep patterns such as sleeping during the day and staying awake all night, insomnia, and/or awakening frequently at night.

Stranger in the Mirror – Signs may include passing a mirror and thinking someone else is in the room, and not realizing that they are the person in the mirror.

Sundowning - Signs may include a state of confusion that typically occurs at the end of the day and into the night, although it can occur at any time. The individual may become demanding, suspicious, disoriented, and/or upset.

Suspicion - Signs may include doubt, mistrust, or misgiving. A person with dementia may doubt the trustworthiness of another person, and believe that their intentions are unreliable, unfavorable, or menacing.

Unusual clothing- Signs may include wearing inappropriate clothing for the weather or occasion, such as a heavy coat in the heat of the summer, or clothing that does not coordinate or match.

Wandering – Signs may include becoming lost even in familiar places, or intrude in inappropriate places. There are many types of wandering including:

- Aimless walking - refers to a type of wandering where a person walks aimlessly around without any specific purpose or goal.
- Checking – refers to a type of wandering where a person is repeatedly seeking the whereabouts of a caregiver or another person.
- Chronic exit seeking – refers to a type of wandering where a person is continuously seeking a way out or away from their current environment. They typically have an agenda or purpose to go somewhere else, such as shopping, to work, to find someone, etc.
- Excessive – refers to a type of wandering where a person is constantly on the move, for an abnormal amount of time, and typically throughout the day.
- Inappropriate purpose – refers to a type of wandering that invades the privacy of another.
- Nighttime walking – refers to a type of wandering in which a person frequently wanders at night.
- Pottering – refers to a type of wandering where a person may walk around and throughout their surroundings possibly trying to accomplish a work related task such as cleaning, laundry, gardening, etc.
- Trailing – refers to a type of wandering where a person follows closely behind another person.
- Withdrawal – Signs may include decreased participation in hobbies, social activities, projects, and/or conversations. A person may ask fewer questions, make less eye contact, and/or may seldom comment or respond to others.

THE STAGES OF PROGRESSION OF ALZHEIMER'S DISEASE AND RELATED DEMENTIAS

Experts have documented common patterns of symptom progression that occur in individuals with brain disease and therefore developed several methods of "stage" categorization based on these patterns. The progression of symptoms generally corresponds to the underlying nerve cell degeneration usually beginning with cells that attack and destroy learning and memory and gradually moves to cells that control all aspects of thinking, judgment, and behavior. The damage eventually spreads to cells that control movement.

Alzheimer's disease typically progresses slowly in three general stages referred to as mild (early-stage), moderate (middle-stage), and severe (late-stage). Since Alzheimer's disease and other dementias affect people in different ways, each person will experience symptoms and/ or progress through the stages differently. Additionally, because the stages may overlap, it may be difficult to definitively place a person in a particular stage. People vary in the length of time spent in any one of the stages, and in which stage the signs and symptoms appear; although, the progression always worsens with time.

These stages describe groups of symptoms that reflect an increase in brain decay, although the rate at which the disease progresses varies. According to the Alzheimer's Association, on average, a person with Alzheimer's disease lives four to eight years after diagnosis, but can live as long as 20 years, depending on other factors.

The stages of Alzheimer's disease described in this section are adapted from the Alzheimer's Association. You can access additional information at http://www.alz.org/alzheimers_disease_stages_of_alzheimers. asp.

The stages provide an overall baseline for assessing how abilities change once symptoms appear. However, changes in the brain related to Alzheimer's disease typically begin years before any signs of the disease are noticed. This time period, which can last for years, is referred to as preclinical Alzheimer's disease.

EARLY STAGE (MILD; 2 – 4 YEARS LEAD-ING UP TO AND INCLUDING DIAGNOSIS)

A person may seem to function quite normally in the earliest stages of the disease. He or she may begin to forget familiar words or the whereabouts of such items as their reading glasses, house keys, etc. He or she may still seem capable of driving, working, and participating in usual social activities with no significantly noticeable changes. Alternatively, friends and family may begin to notice some subtle difficulties. Over time, people with dementia often find it difficult to express themselves and to understand others.

Memory loss is evident in normal aging but differs from memory loss caused by Alzheimer's disease and other related dementias. It is normal for the elderly to experience some rate of decline in cognitive thinking and reasoning abilities. That doesn't necessarily mean they have a brain disease. However, the elderly can still learn and retain new information; whereas, with brain disease, they cannot. An example of normal forgetfulness might be misplacing car keys. Abnormal forgetfulness may be not knowing what the function of your car keys are. Other signs of difficulties associated with brain disease in the early stages (not part of normal aging) may include:

- Difficulty coming up with the right word or name
- Difficulty remembering names when introduced to new people
- Having greater difficulty performing tasks in social or work settings
- Forgetting material that one has just read
- Losing or misplacing a valuable object
- Increasing trouble with planning or organizing
- Repeating familiar words
- Repeating questions, phrases or stories in the same conversation
- Inventing new words to describe familiar objects
- Frequently losing train of thought, or difficulty organizing words logically

- Reverting to speaking in a native language
- Cursing or using offensive words
- Speaking less often
- Relying on non-verbal gestures

Memory loss becomes a problem when it affects the ability to perform everyday tasks. One of the most common early signs of dementia is forgetting recently learned information. While it's perfectly normal to forget appointments, names, or telephone numbers, those with dementia will forget such things more often and not remember them later. They may also experience:

- Challenges in following a plan or familiar recipe
- Trouble keeping track of monthly bills
- Difficulty concentrating
- Taking longer to perform tasks
- Difficulty completing familiar tasks
- Difficulty following directions
- Difficulty understanding large amounts of information
- Difficulty writing
- Difficulty speaking
- Difficulty with rules of syntax and grammar, although the physical ability to speak remains intact
- Difficulty making decisions (often defers to others' choices)
- Difficulty with time orientation
- Experiences long-term and short-term memory loss
- Difficulty understanding rapid speech, or conversation in a noisy environment
- Difficulty coming up with conversation topics
- Difficulty staying on topic
- Difficulty controlling anger
- Increased confusion
- Withdraws from social and mental challenges
- May converse "normally" until a memory lapse occurs
- May become anxious, irritable, or agitated

- May become easily angered when frustrated, tired, rushed, or surprised
- May begin to hoard, check, or search for objects of little value
- May forget to eat, or eat constantly because they forgot they've already eaten, or eat only one kind of food
- Difficulty with judgment, reasoning, and perception
- Difficulty in following a series of steps in the right order
- Loss of spontaneity and initiative

When Alzheimer's disease or other related dementias have been diagnosed early, the loss of abilities is often mild. With a little help, the individual can continue to live independently. However, more often than not, by the time the disease is diagnosed, many of the problems described here may have already progressed to the middle stage.

MIDDLE STAGE (MODERATE; 2 – 10 YEARS AFTER DIAGNOSIS)

During this stage, individuals may have greater difficulty performing normal tasks, but may still remember significant details about their life. Cognitive problems get worse and new ones develop. The damage to the brain has now spread further to areas that control language, reasoning, sensory processing, and conscious thought. The affected regions of the brain continue to shrink (atrophy) resulting in signs and symptoms of the disease becoming more exaggerated and frequent.

Moderate Alzheimer's disease (and associated dementia) is typically the longest stage and can last for many years. As the disease progresses, the person will require a greater level of care.

Some common signs in the middle stage may include an increase in confusing words, getting frustrated or angry, or acting in unexpected ways, such as refusing to bathe. Damage to nerve cells in the brain can make it difficult to express thoughts and perform routine tasks. At this point, symptoms will be noticeable to others and may include:

- Feeling moody or withdrawn, especially in socially or mentally challenging situations
- May become unmannerly, aggressive, or threatening
- Being unable to recall their own address or telephone number or the high school or college from which they graduated
- Confusion about where they are or what day it is
- Difficulty choosing correct clothing
- Trouble controlling bladder and bowels in some individuals
- Changes in sleep patterns, such as sleeping during the day and becoming restless at night
- An increased risk of wandering and becoming lost
- Personality and behavioral changes, including suspiciousness and delusions or compulsive, repetitive behaviors like hand-wringing or tissue shredding. May hear, see, smell, or taste things that aren't really there
- May forget personal history
- Increased memory loss
- Shortened attention span
- Problems recognizing friends and family members
- More difficulty with language, reading, writing, and numbers
- Difficulty organizing thoughts and thinking logically
- Inability to learn new things or to cope with new or unexpected situations
- Loss of impulse control, such as sloppy table manners, undressing at inappropriate times or places, or vulgar language
- Experiencing hallucinations, suspiciousness, irritability, paranoia, and/or delusions
- Repetitive statements, movements, and/or occasional twitches
- Loss of perceptual-motor skills, such as setting the table

- Memory, cognition, and communication difficulties become more severe
- One's personality may change drastically
- Changes in appearance and hygiene as individual becomes less able to take care of themselves
- Increased confusion about time or place orientation
- Increased difficulty in accurately sorting our names with proper faces
- May take others' belongings
- May rummage through things and/or hide things
- May lose track of his/her possessions, or no longer recognizes them
- Difficulty thinking logically or clearly
- May experience a disconnect with reality, such as believing a late spouse is still alive
- May not recognize themselves in the mirror (Stranger in the Mirror syndrome)
- Difficulty performing daily living tasks, such as dressing, bathing, eating, toileting, grooming
- Difficulty finishing sentences
- May revert to native language (first language they learned)
- Changes in sleep patterns; may sleep more often or awake frequently at night
- Increased loss of time and place orientation
- Increased loss of long-term and short-term memory
- Cannot remember 3-item lists or 3-step commands
- Inability to read facial cues, although perception of emotional meaning is retained
- Inability to self-correct
- Loss of ability to speak fluently – will experience more pauses and sentence fragments in conversations
- Inability to finish sentences
- Increased loudness of voice and vocal expression
- May ask fewer questions
- May start fewer conversations
- May make less eye contact

- May withdraw from social situations
- Nouns and proper names may be replaced with pronouns or generic terms such as "thing-a-ma-jig"
- May display inappropriate sexual behavior and may mistake another person for their spouse
- Increased restlessness, pacing, and/or repetitive movements such trying to open doors, and/or tissue shredding
- Increased wandering and chatting to oneself while wandering

END STAGE (SEVERE)

The final stage of Alzheimer's disease and other dementias is the terminal stage. The brain is now severely damaged and most areas of the brain have atrophied, which leads to complete deterioration of the personality. Cognitive symptoms worsen, and the physical symptoms become profound. The loss of brain cells in all parts of the brain leads to lack of functioning in all systems of the body. Earlier stage behaviors disappear, and are replaced by a dulling of the mind and body. Near the end, the person may become completely bedridden and require complete care. The most frequent cause of death is aspiration pneumonia, which develops when a person is not able to swallow properly and ingests food or liquids into the lungs instead of air. During this time, the person with dementia will experience significant losses such as:

- Orientation to time, place, and person
- Loss of awareness of social interaction or expectations
- Loss of desire to communicate
- Loss of ability to form new memories
- Loss of ability to recognize friends and family members
- Loss of ability to understand word meanings
- Loss of grammar and diction, speaks in jargon
- May lose speech altogether

- May become increasingly suspicious, insecure and agitated
- May experience severe sleep disturbances
- May cry out when touched or moved
- May no longer be able to smile
- May appear uncomfortable
- May call or cry out repetitively, groan, or mumble loudly
- May not be able to write or comprehend reading material
- May not be able to control movements and muscles may become rigid
- May be unable to walk without assistance
- May lose the ability to sit
- May lose the ability to hold up their head without support
- May not be able to swallow easily and may choke on food
- Wandering ceases; can't move voluntarily
- May be more vulnerable to infections, especially pneumonia
- May have seizures
- May lose weight
- Skin may become thin and easily tear
- May lose reflexes
- May refuse to eat or drink
- May stop urinating
- May show little response to touch
- Sensory organs may shut down
- May only feel cold and discomfort
- May be severely withdrawn and apathetic
- May exhibit very little communication

CPSIA information can be obtained
at www.ICGtesting.com
Printed in the USA
BVHW080032300921
617786BV00005B/102